LOW HISTAMINE DIET

MAIN COURSE - 60+ Breakfast, Lunch, Dinner and Dessert Recipes for Low Histamine Diet

TABLE OF CONTENTS

purposes solely, and is universal as so. The presentation of the information is without contract or any type of guarantee assurance.

The trademarks that are used are without any consent, and the publication of the trademark is without permission or backing by the trademark owner. All trademarks and brands within this book are for clarifying purposes only and are the owned by the owners themselves, not affiliated with this document.

Introduction

Low histamine recipes for personal enjoyment but also for family enjoyment. You will love them for sure for how easy it is to prepare them.

RAISIN PANCAKES

Serves: **4**

Prep Time: **10** Minutes

Cook Time: **20** Minutes

Total Time: **30** Minutes

INGREDIENTS

- 1 cup whole wheat flour
- ¼ tsp baking soda
- ¼ tsp baking powder
- 1 cup raisins
- 2 eggs
- 1 cup milk

DIRECTIONS

1. In a bowl combine all ingredients together and mix well
2. In a skillet heat olive oil

3. Pour ¼ of the batter and cook each pancake for 1-2 minutes per side

4. When ready remove from heat and serve

Serves: *4*
Prep Time: *10*   Minutes

Cook Time: *30*   Minutes

Total Time: *40*   Minutes

INGREDIENTS

- 1 cup whole wheat flour
- ¼ tsp baking soda
- ¼ tsp goji beri
- 1 cup almonds
- 2 eggs
- 1 cup milk

DIRECTIONS

1. In a bowl combine all ingredients together and mix well
2. In a skillet heat olive oil
3. Pour ¼ of the batter and cook each pancake for 1-2 minutes per side
4. When ready remove from heat and serve

Serves: *4*
Prep Time: *10* Minutes

Cook Time: *20* Minutes

Total Time: *30* Minutes

INGREDIENTS

- 1 cup whole wheat flour
- ¼ tsp baking soda
- ¼ tsp baking powder
- 1 cup mashed banana
- 2 eggs
- 1 cup milk

DIRECTIONS

1. In a bowl combine all ingredients together and mix well
2. In a skillet heat olive oil
3. Pour ¼ of the batter and cook each pancake for 1-2 minutes per side
4. When ready remove from heat and serve

Serves: *4*
Prep Time: *10*   Minutes

Cook Time: *20*   Minutes

Total Time: *30*   Minutes

INGREDIENTS

- 1 cup whole wheat flour
- ¼ tsp baking soda
- ¼ tsp baking powder
- 1 cup mashed mango
- 2 eggs
- 1 cup milk

DIRECTIONS

1. In a bowl combine all ingredients together and mix well
2. In a skillet heat olive oil
3. Pour ¼ of the batter and cook each pancake for 1-2 minutes per side
4. When ready remove from heat and serve

Serves: **4**
Prep Time: **10**   Minutes

Cook Time: **30**   Minutes

Total Time: **40**   Minutes

INGREDIENTS

- **1 cup whole wheat flour**
- **¼ tsp baking soda**
- **¼ tsp baking powder**
- **2 eggs**
- **1 cup milk**
- **1 cup apple**

DIRECTIONS

1. **In a bowl combine all ingredients together and mix well**
2. **In a skillet heat olive oil**
3. **Pour ¼ of the batter and cook each pancake for 1-2 minutes per side**
4. **When ready remove from heat and serve**

Serves: *8-12*
Prep Time: *10*   Minutes

Cook Time: *20*   Minutes

Total Time: *30*   Minutes

INGREDIENTS

- 2 eggs
- 1 tablespoon olive oil
- 1 cup milk
- 2 cups whole wheat flour
- 1 tsp baking soda
- ¼ tsp baking soda
- 1 tsp plum
- 1 tsp cinnamon
- ¼ cup molasses

DIRECTIONS

1. In a bowl combine all dry ingredients
2. In another bowl combine all dry ingredients

3. Combine wet and dry ingredients together

4. Fold in ginger and mix well

5. Pour mixture into 8-12 prepared muffin cups, fill
    2/3 of the cups

6. Bake for 18-20 minutes at 375 F

7. When ready remove from the oven and serve

Serves: *8-12*
Prep Time: *10*   Minutes

Cook Time: *20*   Minutes

Total Time: *30*   Minutes

INGREDIENTS

- 2 eggs
- 1 tablespoon olive oil
- 1 cup milk
- 2 cups whole wheat flour
- 1 tsp baking soda
- ¼ tsp baking soda
- 1 tsp cinnamon
- 1 cup mashed banana

DIRECTIONS

1. In a bowl combine all dry ingredients
2. In another bowl combine all dry ingredients
3. Combine wet and dry ingredients together

4. Fold in mashed banana and mix well
5. Pour mixture into 8-12 prepared muffin cups, fill
   2/3 of the cups
6. Bake for 18-20 minutes at 375 F
7. When ready remove from the oven and serve

Serves: **8-12**
Prep Time: **10** Minutes

Cook Time: **20** Minutes

Total Time: **30** Minutes

INGREDIENTS

- **2 eggs**
- **1 tablespoon olive oil**
- **1 cup milk**
- **2 cups whole wheat flour**
- **1 tsp baking soda**
- **¼ tsp baking soda**
- **1 tsp cinnamon**
- **1 cup acai**

DIRECTIONS

1. **In a bowl combine all dry ingredients**
2. **In another bowl combine all dry ingredients**
3. **Combine wet and dry ingredients together**

4. Fold in blueberries and mix well

5. Pour mixture into 8-12 prepared muffin cups, fill 2/3 of the cups

6. Bake for 18-20 minutes at 375 F

7. When ready remove from the oven and serve

Serves: **8-12**

Prep Time: **10** Minutes

Cook Time: **20** Minutes

Total Time: **30** Minutes

INGREDIENTS

- 2 eggs
- 1 tablespoon olive oil
- 1 cup milk
- 2 cups whole wheat flour
- 1 tsp baking soda
- ¼ tsp baking soda
- 1 tsp cinnamon
- 1 cup apricot

DIRECTIONS

1. In a bowl combine all dry ingredients
2. In another bowl combine all dry ingredients
3. Combine wet and dry ingredients together

4. Fold in strawberries and mix well

5. Pour mixture into 8-12 prepared muffin cups, fill 2/3 of the cups

6. Bake for 18-20 minutes at 375 F

7. When ready remove from the oven and serve

Serves: *8-12*
Prep Time: *10*   Minutes

Cook Time: *20*   Minutes

Total Time: *30*   Minutes

INGREDIENTS

- 2 eggs
- 1 tablespoon olive oil
- 1 cup milk
- 2 cups whole wheat flour
- 1 tsp baking soda
- ¼ tsp baking soda
- 1 cup cherries

DIRECTIONS

1. In a bowl combine all dry ingredients
2. In another bowl combine all dry ingredients
3. Combine wet and dry ingredients together

4. Pour mixture into 8-12 prepared muffin cups, fill 2/3 of the cups

5. Bake for 18-20 minutes at 375 F

6. When ready remove from the oven and serve

Serves: *8-12*
Prep Time: *10*   Minutes

Cook Time: *20*   Minutes

Total Time: *30*   Minutes

INGREDIENTS

- 2 eggs
- 1 tablespoon olive oil
- 1 cup milk
- 2 cups whole wheat flour
- 1 tsp baking soda
- ¼ tsp baking soda
- lemon slices

DIRECTIONS

1. In a bowl combine all dry ingredients
2. In another bowl combine all dry ingredients
3. Combine wet and dry ingredients together

4. Pour mixture into 8-12 prepared muffin cups, fill
    2/3 of the cups

5. Bake for 18-20 minutes at 375 F

6. When ready remove from the oven and serve

Serves: *1*
Prep Time: *5*   Minutes

Cook Time: *10*   Minutes

Total Time: *15*   Minutes

INGREDIENTS

- 2 eggs
- ¼ tsp salt
- ¼ tsp black pepper
- 1 tablespoon olive oil
- ¼ cup cheese
- ¼ cup onion
- ¼ tsp basil

DIRECTIONS

1. In a bowl combine all ingredients together and mix well
2. In a skillet heat olive oil and pour the egg mixture
3. Cook for 1-2 minutes per side

4. When ready remove omelette from the skillet and
    serve

Serves: *1*

Prep Time: *5*   Minutes

Cook Time: *10*   Minutes

Total Time: *15*   Minutes

INGREDIENTS

- 2 eggs
- ¼ tsp salt
- ¼ tsp black pepper
- 1 tablespoon olive oil
- ¼ cup cheese
- ¼ tsp basil
- 1 cup cheese
- 1 cup zucchini

DIRECTIONS

1. In a bowl combine all ingredients together and mix well

2. In a skillet heat olive oil and pour the egg mixture

3. Cook for 1-2 minutes per side

4. When ready remove omelette from the skillet and serve

Serves: *1*
Prep Time: *5*   Minutes

Cook Time: *10*   Minutes

Total Time: *15*   Minutes

INGREDIENTS

- 2 eggs
- ¼ tsp salt
- ¼ tsp black pepper
- 1 tablespoon olive oil
- ¼ cup cheese
- ¼ tsp basil
- 1 cup tomato

DIRECTIONS

1. In a bowl combine all ingredients together and mix well

2. In a skillet heat olive oil and pour the egg mixture

3. Cook for 1-2 minutes per side

4. When ready remove omelette from the skillet and
    serve

Serves: *1*
Prep Time: *5*   Minutes

Cook Time: *10*   Minutes

Total Time: *15*   Minutes

INGREDIENTS

- 2 eggs
- ¼ tsp salt
- ¼ tsp black pepper
- 1 tablespoon olive oil
- ¼ cup cheese
- ¼ tsp basil
- 1 cup cucumber

DIRECTIONS

1. In a bowl combine all ingredients together and mix well

2. In a skillet heat olive oil and pour the egg mixture

3. Cook for 1-2 minutes per side

4. When ready remove omelette from the skillet and
    serve

Serves: *1*
Prep Time: *5*   Minutes

Cook Time: *10*   Minutes

Total Time: *15*   Minutes

INGREDIENTS

- 2 eggs
- ¼ tsp salt
- ¼ tsp black pepper
- 1 tablespoon olive oil
- ¼ cup cheese
- ¼ tsp basil
- 1 cup red bell pepper

DIRECTIONS

1. In a bowl combine all ingredients together and mix well
2. In a skillet heat olive oil and pour the egg mixture
3. Cook for 1-2 minutes per side

4. When ready remove omelette from the skillet and
    serve

Serves: *2*
Prep Time: *10*   Minutes

Cook Time: *5*   Hours

Total Time: *5*   Hours 10 Minutes

INGREDIENTS

- 2 cups milk
- 2 cups water
- 2 cups oats
- ½ cup brown sugar
- 2 tablespoons maple syrup
- 1 tsp cinnamon
- 1 cup blueberries

DIRECTIONS

1. Place all ingredients in a slow cooker, except blueberries and cook on high for 4-5 hours

2. In last 15-20 minutes add the blueberries

3. When ready remove from the slow cooker, add maple syrup and serve

Serves: *1*
Prep Time: *10*   Minutes

Cook Time: *10*   Minutes

Total Time: *20*   Minutes

INGREDIENTS

- 1 cup milk
- 1 cup oats
- 1 tsp cinnamon
- 2 tablespoons brown sugar

DIRECTIONS

1. In a saucepan bring milk to a boil
2. Add cinnamon, oats and cook on low heat for 5-10 minutes
3. In a bowl whisk milk with sugar
4. Add oatmeal to the bowl
5. Sprinkle cinnamon on top and serve

Serves: 2
Prep Time: 5   Minutes

Cook Time: 5   Minutes

Total Time: *10*   Minutes

INGREDIENTS

- 2 slices bread
- 2 tablespoons honey
- 1-2 figs

DIRECTIONS

1. Toast bread and spread honey and layer figs
2. Serve when ready

Serves: *1*
Prep Time: *5*   Minutes

Cook Time: *15*   Minutes

Total Time: *20*   Minutes

INGREDIENTS

- 1 cup coconut milk
- 1 cup oats
- 1 tablespoon coconut flakes
- ½ cup mango

DIRECTIONS

1. In a saucepan bring milk to a boil
2. Stir in oats and simmer on low heat for 5-10 minutes
3. In a skillet toast coconut flakes until golden brown
4. Top oatmeal with mango and roasted coconut flakes

TOMATO FRITATTA

Serves: **2**

Prep Time: **10**   Minutes

Cook Time: **20**   Minutes

Total Time: **30**   Minutes

INGREDIENTS

- ½ lb. tomato
- 1 tablespoon olive oil
- ½ red onion
- ¼ tsp salt
- 2 eggs
- 2 oz. cheddar cheese
- 1 garlic clove
- ¼ tsp dill

DIRECTIONS

1. In a bowl whisk eggs with salt and cheese

2. In a frying pan heat olive oil and pour egg
   mixture

3. Add remaining ingredients and mix well

4. Serve when ready

Serves: **2**
Prep Time: **10** Minutes

Cook Time: **20** Minutes

Total Time: **30** Minutes

INGREDIENTS

- ½ cup yam root
- 1 tablespoon olive oil
- ½ red onion
- ¼ tsp salt
- 2 eggs
- 2 oz. cheddar cheese
- 1 garlic clove
- ¼ tsp dill

DIRECTIONS

1. In a bowl whisk eggs with salt and cheese

2. In a frying pan heat olive oil and pour egg mixture

3. Add remaining ingredients and mix well

4. Serve when ready

Serves: *2*
Prep Time: *10*   Minutes

Cook Time: *20*   Minutes

Total Time: *30*   Minutes

INGREDIENTS

- 1 cup watercress
- 1 tablespoon olive oil
- ½ red onion
- ¼ tsp salt
- 2 eggs
- 2 oz. cheddar cheese
- 1 garlic clove
- ¼ tsp dill

DIRECTIONS

1. In a bowl whisk eggs with salt and cheese

2. In a frying pan heat olive oil and pour egg mixture

3. Add remaining ingredients and mix well

4. Serve when ready

Serves: *2*

Prep Time: *10*   Minutes

Cook Time: *20*   Minutes

Total Time: *30*   Minutes

INGREDIENTS

- 1 cup zucchini
- 1 tablespoon olive oil
- ½ red onion
- ¼ tsp salt
- 2 eggs
- 2 oz. parmesan cheese
- 1 garlic clove
- ¼ tsp dill

DIRECTIONS

1. In a skillet sauté zucchini until tender
2. In a bowl whisk eggs with salt and cheese

3. In a frying pan heat olive oil and pour egg mixture

4. Add remaining ingredients and mix well

5. Serve when ready

Serves: **2**
Prep Time: **10** Minutes

Cook Time: **20** Minutes

Total Time: **30** Minutes

INGREDIENTS

- 1 cup broccoli
- 1 tablespoon olive oil
- ½ red onion
- ¼ tsp salt
- 2 eggs
- 2 oz. cheddar cheese
- 1 garlic clove
- ¼ tsp dill

DIRECTIONS

1. In a skillet sauté broccoli until tender
2. In a bowl whisk eggs with salt and cheese

3. In a frying pan heat olive oil and pour egg
   mixture

4. Add remaining ingredients and mix well

5. Serve when ready

Serves: **2**

Prep Time: **10**   Minutes

Cook Time: **25**   Minutes

Total Time: **35**   Minutes

INGREDIENTS

- **2 chicken breasts**
- **1 tsp salt**
- **6-7 asparagus spears**
- **½ cup mozzarella cheese**
- **2 tsp olive oil**
- **½ cup bread crumbs**

DIRECTIONS

1. **Drizzle olive oil and salt over the chicken breast**
2. **Place the chicken breast in the breadcrumbs bowl and toss well**
3. **Cut the chicken breast and stuff mozzarella inside**

4. Roast chicken breast with asparagus at 400 F for 20-25 minutes

5. When ready remove from the oven and serve

Serves: **2**

Prep Time: **10**   Minutes

Cook Time: **20**   Minutes

Total Time: **30**   Minutes

INGREDIENTS

- 1 cup macaroni
- 1 tablespoon olive oil
- 1 tablespoon all-purpose flour
- 1 tsp salt
- 1 tsp garlic powder
- 1 cup milk
- 1 cup mozzarella cheese
- ½ cup parmesan cheese

DIRECTIONS

1. In a skillet heat olive oil, stir in flour, garlic, salt, milk and cook on low heat
2. Add mozzarella, macaroni and mix well

3. When ready remove from heat and serve with parmesan cheese on top

Serves: *4*
Prep Time: *10*   Minutes

Cook Time: *30*   Minutes

Total Time: *40*   Minutes

INGREDIENTS

- 1 tablespoon olive oil
- ¼ cup red onion
- ½ cup carrots
- 4 cups butternut squash
- 2 cups vegetable stock
- 1 tsp salt

DIRECTIONS

1. In a pot heat olive oil, add onion and cook until tender
2. Add squash and carrots to the pot
3. Add vegetable stock, salt and bring to a boil
4. Simmer on low heat until vegetables are tender

5. Blend the soup until smooth, return to the pot and cook for another 5-10 minutes

6. When ready remove from heat and serve

Serves: **2**
Prep Time: **10** Minutes

Cook Time: **40** Minutes

Total Time: **50** Minutes

INGREDIENTS

- **2 tablespoons butter**
- **1 tablespoon garlic powder**
- **1 tsp rosemary**
- **1 tsp salt**
- **1 cup honey**
- **4 chicken thighs**

DIRECTIONS

1. **In a saucepan melt butter, add garlic, rosemary, salt and simmer on low heat for 30-60 seconds**
2. **Add honey and dip the chicken into the mixture**
3. **Cook for 2-3 minutes, be sure to be well coated**
4. **Transfer to the oven and bake at 400 F for 30-35 minutes**

5. When ready remove from the oven and serve

57

Serves: **2**

Prep Time: **10** Minutes

Cook Time: **30** Minutes

Total Time: **40** Minutes

INGREDIENTS

- **2 cups penne pasta**
- **2 tablespoons butter**
- **1 lb. chicken breast**
- **1 tsp garlic**
- **1 cup canned pumpkin**
- **¼ cup heavy cream**
- **1 tablespoon sage leaves**
- **¼ tsp salt**
- **¼ cup pecans**

DIRECTIONS

1. **Cook pasta and set aside**

2. In a skillet melt butter, add garlic, chicken and
    cook on medium heat until chicken is cooked

3. Add pasta, pumpkin, heavy cream, sage, salt and
    pecans

4. Toss to coat and cook on low heat for 5-10
    minutes

5. When ready remove from the pot and serve

Serves: *6-8*
Prep Time: *10*   Minutes

Cook Time: *15*   Minutes

Total Time: *25*   Minutes

INGREDIENTS

- 1 pizza crust
- ½ cup tomato sauce
- ¼ black pepper
- 1 cup pepperoni slices
- 1 cup mozzarella cheese
- 1 cup olives

DIRECTIONS

1. Spread tomato sauce on the pizza crust
2. Place all the toppings on the pizza crust
3. Bake the pizza at 425 F for 12-15 minutes
4. When ready remove pizza from the oven and serve

Serves:	*6-8*
Prep Time:	*10* Minutes
Cook Time:	*15* Minutes
Total Time:	*25* Minutes

INGREDIENTS

- 1 pizza crust
- ½ cup tomato sauce
- ¼ black pepper
- 1 cup zucchini slices
- 1 cup mozzarella cheese
- 1 cup olives

DIRECTIONS

1. Spread tomato sauce on the pizza crust
2. Place all the toppings on the pizza crust
3. Bake the pizza at 425 F for 12-15 minutes
4. When ready remove pizza from the oven and serve

Serves: 2
Prep Time: 5   Minutes
Cook Time: 5   Minutes
Total Time: *10*   Minutes

INGREDIENTS

- ½ cup olive oil
- 1 lb. cooked steak
- 1 tablespoon taco seasoning
- Juice of 1 lime
- 1 tsp cumin
- 1 head romaine lettuce
- 1 cup corn
- 1 cup beans
- 1 cup tomatoes

DIRECTIONS

1. In a bowl mix all ingredients and mix well
2. Serve with dressing

Serves: **2**

Prep Time: **5**   Minutes

Cook Time: **5**   Minutes

Total Time: **10**   Minutes

INGREDIENTS

- 2 cups kale
- 1 tablespoon hemp seeds
- 1 cucumber
- 1 tsp honey
- 1 tsp olive oil
- 1 handful parsley

DIRECTIONS

1. In a bowl mix all ingredients and mix well
2. Serve with dressing

Serves: 2
Prep Time: 5   Minutes

Cook Time: 5   Minutes

Total Time: *10*   Minutes

INGREDIENTS

- 1 cup cauliflower
- 1 cup broccoli
- 1 cup brussels sprouts
- 1 cup red bell pepper
- 1 cup squash
- 1 tablespoon olive oil

DIRECTIONS

1. In a bowl mix all ingredients and mix well
2. Serve with dressing

Serves: **2**
Prep Time: **5**   Minutes

Cook Time: **5**   Minutes

Total Time: **10**   Minutes

INGREDIENTS

- ½ cauliflower florets
- 1 cup pumpkin
- 1 cup Brussel sprouts
- 1 cup quinoa
- 1 tablespoon olive oil

DIRECTIONS

1. In a bowl mix all ingredients and mix well
2. Serve with dressing

Serves: 2
Prep Time: 5   Minutes
Cook Time: 5   Minutes
Total Time: *10*   Minutes

INGREDIENTS

- 1 cooked duck breast
- ½ lb. Brussel sprouts
- 1 cup broccoli florets
- 1 apple
- 3 oz. blueberries
- 1 tsp olive oil
- 1 cup blueberry salad dressing

DIRECTIONS

1. In a bowl mix all ingredients and mix well
2. Serve with dressing

Serves: *2*

Prep Time: *5*   Minutes

Cook Time: *5*   Minutes

Total Time: *10*   Minutes

INGREDIENTS

- ½ lb. Brussels sprouts
- 1 cup cauliflower florets
- ½ lb. carrot
- 2 oz. lettuce
- 3 oz. cooked breast chicken
- 1 tsp olive oil

DIRECTIONS

1. In a bowl mix all ingredients and mix well
2. Serve with dressing

Serves: 2
Prep Time: 5   Minutes

Cook Time: 5   Minutes

Total Time: *10*   Minutes

INGREDIENTS

- 1 tablespoon olive oil
- 1 tablespoon apple cider vinegar
- 1 tablespoon lemon juice
- 1 tsp turmeric
- 1 clove garlic
- 1 tsp salt

DIRECTIONS

1. In a bowl mix all ingredients and mix well
2. Serve with dressing

Serves: **2**

Prep Time: **5** Minutes

Cook Time: **5** Minutes

Total Time: **10** Minutes

INGREDIENTS

- 2 red chicory
- 2 fennel bulbs
- ½ cup watercress
- 2 garlic cloves
- 1 tablespoon olive oil

DIRECTIONS

1. In a bowl mix all ingredients and mix well
2. Serve with dressing

Serves: **2**
Prep Time: **5**   Minutes

Cook Time: **5**   Minutes

Total Time: **10**   Minutes

INGREDIENTS

- **1 fennel bulb**
- **1 tablespoon lemon juice**
- **¼ cup olive oil**
- **1 tsp mint**
- **1 tsp onion**

DIRECTIONS

1. **In a bowl mix all ingredients and mix well**
2. **Serve with dressing**

Serves: **2**
Prep Time: **5**   Minutes

Cook Time: **5**   Minutes

Total Time: ***10***   Minutes

INGREDIENTS

- 2 lb. sweet potatoes
- ¼ cup olive oil
- 2 tablespoons lemon juice
- ¼ cup scallions
- ¼ cup cilantro
- ¼ tsp salt

DIRECTIONS

1. In a bowl mix all ingredients and mix well
2. Serve with dressing

CAULIFLOWER RECIPE

Serves: *6-8*
Prep Time: *10*   Minutes

Cook Time: *15*   Minutes

Total Time: *25*   Minutes

INGREDIENTS

- 1 pizza crust
- ½ cup tomato sauce
- ¼ black pepper
- 1 cup cauliflower
- 1 cup mozzarella cheese
- 1 cup olives

DIRECTIONS

1. Spread tomato sauce on the pizza crust
2. Place all the toppings on the pizza crust
3. Bake the pizza at 425 F for 12-15 minutes

4. When ready remove pizza from the oven and
    serve

Serves: *6-8*
Prep Time: *10*   Minutes

Cook Time: *15*   Minutes

Total Time: *25*   Minutes

INGREDIENTS

- 1 pizza crust
- ½ cup tomato sauce
- ¼ black pepper
- 1 cup broccoli
- 1 cup mozzarella cheese
- 1 cup olives

DIRECTIONS

1. Spread tomato sauce on the pizza crust
2. Place all the toppings on the pizza crust
3. Bake the pizza at 425 F for 12-15 minutes
4. When ready remove pizza from the oven and serve

Serves: *6-8*
Prep Time: *10*   Minutes

Cook Time: *15*   Minutes

Total Time: *25*   Minutes

INGREDIENTS

- 1 pizza crust
- ½ cup tomato sauce
- ¼ black pepper
- 1 cup pepperoni slices
- 1 cup tomatoes
- 6-8 ham slices
- 1 cup mozzarella cheese
- 1 cup olives

DIRECTIONS

1. Spread tomato sauce on the pizza crust
2. Place all the toppings on the pizza crust
3. Bake the pizza at 425 F for 12-15 minutes

4. When ready remove pizza from the oven and
    serve

Serves: *4*

Prep Time: *10*   Minutes

Cook Time: *20*   Minutes

Total Time: *30*   Minutes

INGREDIENTS

- 1 tablespoon olive oil
- 1 lb. mushrooms
- ¼ red onion
- ½ cup all-purpose flour
- ¼ tsp salt
- ¼ tsp pepper
- 1 can vegetable broth
- 1 cup heavy cream

DIRECTIONS

1. In a saucepan heat olive oil and sauté mushrooms until tender
2. Add remaining ingredients to the saucepan and bring to a boil

3. When all the vegetables are tender transfer to a blender and blend until smooth

4. Pour soup into bowls, garnish with parsley and serve

Serves: *4*

Prep Time: *10* Minutes

Cook Time: *20* Minutes

Total Time: *30* Minutes

INGREDIENTS

- 1 tablespoon olive oil
- ¼ red onion
- ½ cup all-purpose flour
- ¼ tsp salt
- ¼ tsp pepper
- 1 can vegetable broth
- 1 cup heavy cream

DIRECTIONS

1. In a saucepan heat olive oil and sauté onion until tender
2. Add remaining ingredients to the saucepan and bring to a boil

3. When all the vegetables are tender transfer to a blender and blend until smooth

4. Pour soup into bowls, garnish with parsley and serve

Serves: *4*

Prep Time: *10* Minutes

Cook Time: *20* Minutes

Total Time: *30* Minutes

INGREDIENTS

- 1 tablespoon olive oil
- 1 lb. green pepper
- ¼ red onion
- ½ cup all-purpose flour
- ¼ tsp salt
- ¼ tsp pepper
- 1 can vegetable broth
- 1 cup heavy cream

DIRECTIONS

1. In a saucepan heat olive oil and sauté green pepper until tender
2. Add remaining ingredients to the saucepan and bring to a boil

3. When all the vegetables are tender transfer to a blender and blend until smooth

4. Pour soup into bowls, garnish with parsley and serve

Serves: *4*

Prep Time: *10* Minutes

Cook Time: *20* Minutes

Total Time: *30* Minutes

INGREDIENTS

- 1 tablespoon olive oil
- 1 lb. pumpkin
- ¼ red onion
- ½ cup all-purpose flour
- ¼ tsp salt
- ¼ tsp pepper
- 1 can vegetable broth
- 1 cup heavy cream

DIRECTIONS

1. In a saucepan heat olive oil and sauté carrots until tender
2. Add remaining ingredients to the saucepan and bring to a boil

3. When all the vegetables are tender transfer to a blender and blend until smooth

4. Pour soup into bowls, garnish with parsley and serve

Serves: *4*

Prep Time: *10* Minutes

Cook Time: *20* Minutes

Total Time: *30* Minutes

INGREDIENTS

- 1 tablespoon olive oil
- 1 lb. swiss chard
- ¼ red onion
- ½ cup all-purpose flour
- ¼ tsp salt
- ¼ tsp pepper
- 1 can vegetable broth
- 1 cup heavy cream

DIRECTIONS

1. In a saucepan heat olive oil and sauté potatoes until tender
2. Add remaining ingredients to the saucepan and bring to a boil

3. When all the vegetables are tender transfer to a blender and blend until smooth

4. Pour soup into bowls, garnish with parsley and serve

APPLE-GINGER SMOOTHIE

Serves: *1*

Prep Time: *5* Minutes

Cook Time: *5* Minutes

Total Time: *10* Minutes

INGREDIENTS

- 1 apple
- 1 cup almond milk
- 1 cup kale
- 1 tsp ginger

DIRECTIONS

1. In a blender place all ingredients and blend until smooth
2. Pour smoothie in a glass and serve

Serves: *1*
Prep Time: **5**   Minutes

Cook Time: **5**   Minutes

Total Time: **10**   Minutes

INGREDIENTS

- 1 cucumber
- 1 pomegranate
- 1 cup ice
- 1 cup almond milk

DIRECTIONS

1. **In a blender place all ingredients and blend until smooth**
2. **Pour smoothie in a glass and serve**

Serves: *1*
Prep Time: *5*   Minutes

Cook Time: *5*   Minutes

Total Time: *10*   Minutes

INGREDIENTS

- 1 mango
- 1 cup strawberries
- 1 cup coconut milk
- 1 cup ice

DIRECTIONS

1. In a blender place all ingredients and blend until smooth
2. Pour smoothie in a glass and serve

Serves: *1*
Prep Time: *5*   Minutes

Cook Time: *5*   Minutes

Total Time: *10*   Minutes

INGREDIENTS

- 1 cup caramel powder
- 1 cup almond milk
- 1 tsp cinnamon

DIRECTIONS

1. In a blender place all ingredients and blend until smooth
2. Pour smoothie in a glass and serve

Serves: *1*

Prep Time: **5**   Minutes

Cook Time: **5**   Minutes

Total Time: **10**   Minutes

INGREDIENTS

- 1 cup blueberries
- 1 cup water
- 2 basil leaves
- ½ cup coconut milk
- 1 tablespoon peanut butter

DIRECTIONS

1. In a blender place all ingredients and blend until smooth
2. Pour smoothie in a glass and serve

Serves: *1*

Prep Time: *5* Minutes

Cook Time: *5* Minutes

Total Time: *10* Minutes

INGREDIENTS

- 1 cup blueberries
- 1 cup cauliflower
- 1 cup vanilla yoghurt
- 1 cup protein powder

DIRECTIONS

1. In a blender place all ingredients and blend until smooth
2. Pour smoothie in a glass and serve

Serves: *1*
Prep Time: *5*   Minutes

Cook Time: *5*   Minutes

Total Time: *10*   Minutes

INGREDIENTS

- 1 nectarine
- 2 oz. cauliflower
- 2 oz. swiss chard
- 1 tablespoon almond butter

DIRECTIONS

1. In a blender place all ingredients and blend until smooth
2. Pour smoothie in a glass and serve

Serves: *1*
Prep Time: *5*   Minutes

Cook Time: *5*   Minutes

Total Time: *10* Minutes

INGREDIENTS

- 2 oz. baby spinach
- 1 cucumber
- 1 apple
- ¼ avocado
- 1 tsp ginger

DIRECTIONS

1. In a blender place all ingredients and blend until smooth
2. Pour smoothie in a glass and serve

Serves: *1*
Prep Time: *5*   Minutes

Cook Time: *5*   Minutes

Total Time: *10*   Minutes

INGREDIENTS

- 2 carrots
- 1 red beet
- ½ tomato
- One handful of watercress
- ½ cup ice

DIRECTIONS

1. In a blender place all ingredients and blend until smooth
2. Pour smoothie in a glass and serve

Serves: *1*
Prep Time: **5**   Minutes

Cook Time: **5**   Minutes

Total Time: *10*   Minutes

INGREDIENTS

- 1 cup broccoli
- 2 celery sticks
- 1 fennel bulb
- 1 cucumber
- 1 cup ice

DIRECTIONS

1. In a blender place all ingredients and blend until smooth
2. Pour smoothie in a glass and serve

THANK YOU FOR READING THIS BOOK!